God's Pathway to Healing

HEART

BOOKS BY REGINALD B. CHERRY, M.D.

GOD'S PATHWAY TO HEALING:

Bone Health

Diabetes

Digestion

Heart

Herbs That Heal

Joints and Arthritis

The Immune System

Memory and Mental Acuity

Menopause

Prostate

Vision

Vitamins and Supplements

Dr. Cherry's Little Instruction Book

God's Pathway to Healing

HEART

by

Reginald B. Cherry, M.D.

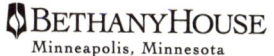
Minneapolis, Minnesota

God's Pathway to Healing: Heart
Copyright © 2003
Reginald B. Cherry, M.D.

Page 160 is a continuation of the copyright page.

Manuscript prepared by Rick Killian, Killian Creative, Boulder, Colorado. *www.killiancreative.com*

Cover design by Danielle White

Note: The directions given in this book are in no way to be considered a substitute for consultation with your own physician.

All rights reserved. No part of this publication may be reproduced, stored in a retrieval system, or transmitted in any form or by any means—electronic, mechanical, photocopying, recording, or otherwise—without the prior written permission of the publisher and copyright owners.

Published by Bethany House Publishers
11400 Hampshire Avenue South
Bloomington, Minnesota 55438

Bethany House Publishers is a Division of
Baker Book House Company, Grand Rapids, Michigan.

Printed in the United States of America

ISBN 0-7642-2814-5

CONTENTS

Introduction 9

1. Facing the "Goliath" of
   Heart Disease 17

2. Understanding the Giant of
   Cardiovascular Disease 31
   CVD's Most Common Foothold:
      Atherosclerosis................. 36
   The Sudden Killer: Heart Attacks 42
   Taking on Goliath 50

3. The Five Smooth Stones That Will
   Defeat Cardiovascular Disease...... 53
   (1) Stop Smoking and Avoid
      Secondhand Smoke 56

(2) Exercise and Control Weight 59
   Determine Your Safe Heart-Rate Range 62
(3) Adopt a Low-Fat, Low-Cholesterol, Low-Sodium, High-Fiber Diet ... 63
   The Mediterranean Diet 64
   Soybeans: The Plant Kingdom's Best Protein Substitute 76
   Addressing Cholesterol Specifically 80
   High Cholesterol May Be a Result of Low Thyroid Output 83
(4) Begin a Basic Daily Vitamin and Nutritional Supplement Program   84
(5) Use Other Natural Compounds That Specifically Address Cardiovascular Disease 87
   Natural Compounds to Address Cardiovascular Disease in General 88
   L-Arginine 88

Aspirin 89
B-Vitamins and Betaine 90
Coenzyme Q10 (ubiquinone). 91
Docosahexaenoic acid (DHA) and
    eicosapentaenoic acid (EPA) 92
Garlic bulb extract 93
Green tea extract 94
Grape-seed and grape-skin extracts 95
Hawthorn 97
Magnesium 98
Notoginseng 99
Policosanol. 99
Taurine. 102
Tocotrienols. 102
Cardiovascular Disease Can Be
Beaten 103
4. Specifically Combating Hypertension
and Heart Arrhythmia 107
    Natural Compounds to Combat

- Hypertension 108
  - Potassium 109
  - Polyphenols 110
  - Magnesium.................. 111
- Natural Compounds to Combat Heart Arrhythmia 112
- God Designed These Compounds to Work Together 115
5. Your Daily Walk on the Pathway to a Healthy Heart and Cardiovascular System 119
  - God Has a Unique Pathway to Cardiovascular Health for You 128
- Endnotes........................... 131
- Reginald B. Cherry, M.D.—
  - A Medical Doctor's Testimony..... 135
- About the Author 141
- Resources Available From
  - Reginald B. Cherry Ministries, Inc. 143
- Become a Pathway to Healing Partner 157

INTRODUCTION

In the last century or so, heart disease has gone from being a relatively minor occurrence to the number one killer in the Western nations. More people die of heart disease than of the next five leading causes of death *combined*. Between 40 and 50 percent in these countries—that is, nearly one of every two people—will die from some form of cardiovascular disease. The Bible tells us, "The life of the flesh is in the blood" (Leviticus 17:11). When we begin to cut off the flow of that blood, life starts dwindling. The end result is always death, unless we can reverse this trend by strengthening our heart and keeping our blood flowing without hindrance.

Cardiovascular disease has been called the "silent killer" because it can have few signs or symptoms until it strikes and then can erupt in a heart attack, often causing death within four or five minutes. Heart attacks cause more fatalities in the United States and Western Europe than any other illness, though heart attacks rarely happen without some other form of cardiovascular disease—such as hardening or clogging of the arteries or high blood pressure—having been present for a period of time beforehand. This is one reason why regular checkups with a health professional are so important—early detection of cardiovascular problems is vital to preventing coronary heart disease events. Recent studies are finding that signs of heart disease are showing up much earlier than mid-life—which is when most begin to look for them—and, in fact, are even present in preteen children and adolescents. Cardiovascular disease is actually the number two killer (behind accidents) of children under the age of fifteen. Heart disease is also an equal-opportunity killer, being the leading cause of death for men and women alike as well as for every race living in the industrialized nations. Because of these facts, we each need to know what cardiovascular disease is and how to prevent it.

The study of cardiovascular disease has become an area of major focus in recent decades. Though there is now a better understanding of what causes certain cardiovascular diseases and how they can be treated with natural compounds, ranging from grape-seed extract to CoQ10 and policosanol, the bulk of the research still points to controlling what we consume as the best means of prevention. Overcoming the habit of smoking in addition to eliminating excessive fat and cholesterol from our diet are the main keys. Because heart disease can strike suddenly and kill quickly, it is important to take the necessary steps to prevent it rather than try to cure it once it has developed. However, if you have suffered a coronary heart disease event, research now points to some things that can prevent your having another event and even reversing some of the damage that caused it in the first place.

Proverbs 4:23 (NKJV) instructs us: "Keep your heart with all diligence, for out of it spring the issues of life." Heart and cardiovascular disease are not only deadly but also affect all other areas of our physical well-being. The poor blood flow caused by a weak heart or hardening and clogging of the arteries is linked to everything from memory loss and poor concentration to pain in the legs and joints to sexual performance to the proper functioning of the immune system. Just as the Bible speaks of the heart as the center of our spiritual lives, so it is the center of a healthy mind and body.

The problems we are speaking of are *not* part of God's plan for our lives. He said He would keep sickness from the midst of us by blessing our food and water. (See Exodus 23:25–26.) He also said He would satisfy us with long life (see Psalm 91:16) and that Jesus came that we might have life and have it more abundantly (see John 10:10). The good news is that God has a pathway to a healthy heart for you and your loved ones. I pray that the following chapters will help you to find it and to follow it.

—Reginald B. Cherry, M.D.

Chapter 1

FACING THE "GOLIATH" OF HEART DISEASE

Chapter 1

FACING THE "GOLIATH" OF HEART DISEASE

"Don't be impressed with your own wisdom. Instead, fear the LORD and turn your back on evil. Then you will gain renewed health and vitality" (Proverbs 3:7–8 NLT).

According to recent statistics released by the American Heart Association, cardiovascular disease kills nearly 950,000 Americans every year (of these, almost 150,000 are under the age of sixty-five) and affects roughly 61.8 million—costing us approximately $352 billion annually to treat. It has been the leading killer in the United States every year since 1900, except at the height of WWI in 1918. Nearly 2,600 Americans die of cardiovascular disease every day, which is an average of one death every thirty-three seconds. It claims more lives than the next five leading causes of death *combined:* which are cancer, chronic lower respiratory disease, accidents, diabetes mellitus, and influenza/pneumonia. One in five Americans presently has some form of cardiovascular disease, and as many as one of every two of us will eventually die because of it.[1] It is evident that in cardiovascular disease we face a giant of epidemic proportions.

Yet when David faced his giant, Goliath,

Facing the "Goliath" of Heart Disease

he did not fear but rather looked to the Lord for victory. I believe that his is the example we should take as we face the Goliath of cardiovascular disease. We need not fear, because we can turn to God's Word and wisdom for victory.

Heart disease has not always been the killer it is today in the United States, nor is it as lethal in other countries, especially lesser-developed countries. In places where the diet is more natural and less processed and fatty, heart disease hardly exists. You will also find that people are less sedentary in these places because cars and television are not so common—thus, they spend more time outdoors and walking to get from place to place. It seems in our rush for progress, we have lost a few basics that could literally cost us our lives. As in every area of life, we need to look to the Bible for answers.

Proverbs 3:1–4 (NLT) tells us,

> Never forget the things I have taught you. Store my commands in your heart for they will give you a long, satisfying life. Never let loyalty and kindness get away from you! Wear them like a necklace; write them deep within your heart. Then you will find favor with both God and people, and you will gain a good reputation.

Then in verse 5, it says, "Trust in the Lord with all your heart; do not depend on your own understanding."

The lifestyle we live today that is leading to cardiovascular disease is one that is imbedded in our culture and in our habits—in our "own understanding," if you will. This understanding dictates our wants and desires. And these wants and desires will have to undergo a radical change if we are to defeat the giant of heart disease. Look what Proverbs 3:6–8 (NLT) goes on to say with regard to this: "Seek his will in all you do, and he will direct your paths. Don't be impressed with your own wisdom. Instead, fear the LORD and turn your back on evil. Then you will gain renewed health and vitality."

Of course, we aren't saying that poor eating habits and lack of regular exercise are evil, but if we look closely at the Scriptures, we will see that our habits today are very different from those outlined in the Old Testament laws or those seen in the days Jesus walked on the earth. Some may say, "But the Bible doesn't advocate exercise. Jesus never told His disciples to run forty-five minutes, four times a week!" That's true, but if we look at the lifestyle then, we will see that Jesus and His disciples walked everywhere—even to towns fifty miles away! He didn't need to tell them to jog in order to get the necessary exercise. Nor do we hear Jesus say much about what they should eat or not eat; they were already following the Jewish food laws of the Old Testament, and they were eating a Mediterranean diet because of where they lived—one that science today is finding to be one of the healthiest in the world. Jesus' focus was on teaching about His spiritual kingdom, not our earthly one. What we eat has nothing to do with being righteous before God. However, I believe it has a great deal to do with having the abundant life or "life in all its fullness" that Jesus promised (see John 10:10).

The Bible contains moral laws that we need to follow, but it is also filled with principles that, though not necessary for righteousness, lead to blessing. Otherwise, our Christian walk would be over once we were born again and became part of Jesus' righteousness before God. Our names at that point are written in the Lamb's Book of Life, and we are heaven bound, but is that all there is to it? *No.* We have much to learn and walk out for our testimony and for the glory of God.

You may respond, "Well, I'm under the new covenant, and I don't have to keep those laws." That may be true. As a Christian, you are not obligated to keep the laws of the old covenant in order to be righteous before God. The Israelites had to keep the law to be righteous because their righteousness was dependent upon the law. Of course, they found it impossible to keep the whole letter of the law, and that's why a priest had to go in once a year and make atonement for them. But the Bible says that Jesus is the end of the law for righteousness. In other words, He ended the ceremonial law God's people had to follow to be righteous. Now we live by the law of love that He has put directly into our hearts, but this does not do away with the blessing of the dietary and moral laws. We still keep the Ten Commandments, which bring blessing on our nation and our communities, and I believe that if we retain the essence of the dietary laws, we will still receive the blessing of health that He promised in Exodus 23:25–26: "And ye shall serve the LORD your God, and he shall bless thy bread, and thy water; and I will take sickness away from the midst of thee. There shall nothing cast their young, nor be barren, in thy land: the number of thy days I will fulfil." In other words, He will bless our food, and we will stay healthy.

You can eat a high-fat, fast-food hamburger—which violates Leviticus 3:17: "Eat neither fat nor blood" and Leviticus 7:23: "Ye shall eat no manner of fat"—and still be righteous before God. And you may see God a whole lot sooner if you do that often enough, because eating saturated animal fat regularly has natural consequences (sickness and disease) that are not part of God's plan for healthy living and definitely are not His pathway to healing cardiovascular disease.

All of us as human beings have a pathway to healing, and often it will involve something natural. I base this on John 9:6–7, where Jesus, through natural means, allowed healing to flow through the cleansing of mud and saliva to restore sight to a blind man. Jesus "spat on the ground, and made clay of the spittle, and he anointed the eyes of the blind man with the clay," but this touch of Jesus alone did not heal him. It was not until the blind man obeyed Jesus' words, "Go, wash in the pool of Siloam," that the man received his sight.

In essence, Jesus said, "There's a path. I want you to follow that path and find a pool called Siloam, and when you reach that pool, reach down and wash the clay and the spittle from your eyes, and you shall receive your sight." The healing came because the man obeyed God's word to him.

If we are willing to open ourselves to

God's Word and wisdom today, I believe He has a pathway to healing and health for us. We will probably have to change our lifestyles somewhat—especially our diet and exercise habits—but aren't those changes worth the blessing of health we will reap?

We need not fear the giant of heart disease. If we will seek after God's pathway to defeating it, we can say—just as David did—"Let no man's heart fail because of this giant.... The Lord will deliver me out of his hand" (1 Samuel 17:32, 37, paraphrased).

Chapter 2

UNDERSTANDING THE GIANT OF CARDIOVASCULAR DISEASE

Chapter 2

UNDERSTANDING THE GIANT OF CARDIOVASCULAR DISEASE

Cardiovascular disease (CVD) includes all the major illnesses that affect the cardiovascular system, which is made up of

(1) the heart;
(2) the blood;
(3) the arteries (that carry the blood away from the heart and to body tissues);
(4) the capillaries (the weblike network of smaller vessels with thin walls

that feed the nutrients in the blood to the body tissues);

(5) the veins (that carry the blood back from the body tissues to the heart).

The primary diseases in this category are

- Atherosclerosis (a form of arteriosclerosis—which is the general term for hardening or clogging of the arteries—in which pulpy, lipid-containing plaques [called atheroma] cause the arteries to harden, thicken, and sometimes clog)
- Hypertension (high blood pressure)
- Coronary artery disease (also called coronary heart disease; when arteriosclerosis affects the arteries that feed the heart muscle)
- Carotid artery disease (when arterioscle-

rosis affects the arteries that feed the brain)
- Peripheral artery disease (when arteriosclerosis affects the arteries that feed the "peripheral" parts of the body—the legs in particular)
- Heart disease (which we will define as diseases affecting the heart directly for our discussion here, though "heart disease" and "cardiovascular disease" are often used interchangeably—this can be anything from arrhythmic heartbeats to congestive heart failure)

Although these diseases can be distinguished and studied separately, they are often as interconnected as the cardiovascular system itself—one leading to the next and then accelerating another. There is rarely any sign or symptom of any of these illnesses until there is a coronary heart disease event, such as chest pains (angina pectoris) or a heart attack (a myocardial infarction), although having regular checkups can diagnose indications that one or more of these diseases may be developing.

While the likelihood of coronary heart disease events do increase with age, heart disease is not a part of aging but rather the result of a number of factors over time. The mortality rates of cardiovascular disease in many lesser-developed countries are actually much lower, even among the elderly; just as the mortality rate of cardiovascular disease was much lower in the Western world before the turn of the twentieth century—while it is number one today, it wasn't even in the top ten at that time.[1] Most likely the primary reasons for this are:

(1) Our diets are higher in animal/dairy fats, cholesterol, salt, and processed, refined foods and lower in fiber than those of other cultures and our own a century ago.
(2) We live more sedentary lives and are also more overweight.
(3) We breathe in more pollutants, whether it is through smoking ourselves, breathing secondhand smoke, or the general air pollution that is common in our cities.

While there are several secondary causes in addition to these—among which are family history, obesity, diabetes, and nutritional deficiencies of certain key vitamins, minerals, and fatty acids—addressing these three main causes will answer many of our questions about how cardiovascular disease begins and how it develops.

CVD's Most Common Foothold: Atherosclerosis

In general, the most common start of cardiovascular disease is atherosclerosis. This is when deposits of pulpy, acellular, lipid-containing plaques—oxidized low-density lipoprotein (LDL) cholesterol is the most common of these; sometimes calcium is in it as well—begin to collect inside the walls of the blood vessels, particularly the arteries. To understand exactly what that does, we have to first understand a little more about the functions and anatomy of the arteries.

Arteries are made up of several layers, but to simplify our discussion, we will focus on the main three:

(1) the adventitia (the outside of the blood vessel);
(2) the elastic membrane or muscles that make up the center of the arteries;
(3) the endothelium (the interior lining of the arteries and veins).

When the heart pumps, the entire circular wall of the artery expands like an elastic balloon, absorbing the shock of the pulsation. This is the high point in a blood pressure reading, called the systolic blood pressure. When the heart rests, the arteries contract again, forcing the blood farther along toward the body tissues it is meant to feed. This is the low point in the blood pressure reading, or the diastolic blood pressure. Normal blood pressure is 100/70 to 135/85, the first number representing the pressure when the heart pumps and the vessels expand, and the second when the heart rests and the arteries constrict. If the walls of the arteries did not constrict, the blood pressure would be 0; so a normal blood pressure reading would be something like 110/0, but as they do constrict between heartbeats, a steady—though lesser—pressure is maintained and the blood continues to flow. The elasticity of these vessels is key to not overworking the heart to and keeping it healthy.

What atherosclerosis does is deposit its fatty plaques somewhere within the wall of the artery, between the endothelium and the adventitia. In fact, these plaque deposits (called atheromas) are most commonly in the adventitia and are missed completely by traditional angiograms (a test used to uncover artery diseases).[2] This is most common in areas where the endothelium has been damaged. This damage is often caused by free radicals—renegade O_1 oxygen molecules that are missing an electron. They wander our systems looking to "tear" one away from somewhere else, thus damaging the cells from which they steal this electron (healthy oxygen molecules are O_2 molecules and can be absorbed by our systems as a nutrient). Cigarette smoke is a common pollutant that causes free radicals.

These deposits are not evenly distributed, and they make rough spots and bulges in the artery walls. The more of these "rough spots" that form, the harder our arteries become, losing their elasticity. As these fatty plaques grow, they also shrink the channel within the arteries through which the blood flows. Blood flow is thus reduced, and the heart has to work harder to pump enough nutrient-laden blood to the various parts of our bodies. The long-term results of this process are numerous: high blood pressure (anything over 140/90); any of the various artery diseases, depending on which areas are affected the most by these plaque buildups; chest pains; bulging or bubbling of the arteries (aneurysms); various other problems in our bodies because of the reduction of blood flow; and enlargement of the heart, which will eventually lead to congestive heart failure (when the heart muscle literally wears out and dies—the only solution to which is a heart transplant).

Understanding the Giant of Cardiovascular Disease

Though the worst effects of atherosclerosis don't usually appear until around middle-age, indications are that the disease actually begins much earlier. One study looked at heart transplant donors (those who had volunteered the use of their organs to save the lives of others in the event of their own death from an accident). In looking at each decade of life, they found the following percentages had hardening of the arteries:

- 17 percent of those under the age of 20
- 37 percent of those in their 20s
- 60 percent of those in their 30s
- 71 percent of those in their 40s
- 85 percent of those in their 50s

Other research has confirmed that junk-food diets and lack of exercise in children are directly associated with the development of atherosclerosis starting at a young age. Diet and exercise do matter, even in childhood. The American Heart Association has recently released guidelines for addressing atherosclerosis in children.[3]

THE SUDDEN KILLER: HEART ATTACKS

Because atherosclerosis develops over time, for decades doctors thought they had the cause of heart attacks figured out: it was simply a matter of a plumbing problem. Just as old pipes in a house fill with mineral deposits and then are clogged, so it was thought that our coronary arteries (those that directly feed the heart muscle) get filled up with cholesterol and calcium and then shut off the flow of blood to the heart, causing a myocardial infarction (MI)—which is the technical name for a heart attack or a "coronary." Because doctors believed this was a gradual process, angina symptoms (chest pain) were seen as indicators of a heart attack that was months or years away.

Yet as heart disease came under more and more scrutiny, evidence arose that showed this theory was flawed somewhere. Heart attacks were being caused by blockages in the arteries that had been relatively clear before (approximately 10 to 30 percent blocked) and caused no chest pain; while areas that were as much as 80 to 90 percent blocked—though they did cause chest pain—were not causing heart attacks. So it appears that the scaly calcium that slowly hardens and/or thickens our arteries is not the major cause of heart attacks. Instead, it has to be something that acts quickly and blocks the entire coronary artery in a very short time.

What researchers now believe happens is that a soft, fatty plaque that deposits inside the artery walls can suddenly cause a rupture in the endothelium (the innermost layer of a blood vessel) and cause a clot that blocks the artery in a matter of minutes. It appears that not all plaques are the same. Though all plaques are in most cases made up of some mixture of cholesterol, fats, fibrous tissue, and white blood cells, this mixture varies widely. While some plaques are firmer and more stable, others are softer. The plaque that is apparently causing heart attacks has more cholesterol and fats in its center, which makes it much softer—called "vulnerable plaque"—and can cause inflammation in the side of the artery just as an infection does

Understanding the Giant of Cardiovascular Disease

---

below the skin. Then if the endothelium is unhealthy because it is brittle or "shredded" by impurities in the blood, it bursts through and begins to ooze into the flow of blood. The body interprets this as a cut in the vessel, and the platelets that are responsible for blood clotting rush to the area to wall it off, just as they do when a cut breaks your skin and they rush to block the blood flow to keep you from bleeding to death. Except in the former case, they are walling off the blood flow within a closed artery, and the platelets clump together, forming a barrier to the blood passing through the vessel rather than between the break in the vessel and the outside.

Now, if this process works to merely put a fibrous cap on the inner surface of the artery and seal the rupture, things can go on as normal for some time. The clot may only grow to a certain size, partially blocking the blood vessel and causing some chest pain. But if it builds larger than that, the chest pain will become more severe, radiating out from the middle of the chest (usually to the left side and many times down the arm). Either could be the beginning of a heart attack, signaling that the person should be rushed to the hospital.

There is evidence that high homocysteine levels act as a catalyst in the process, which is why homocysteine is considered a risk for CVD independent of other factors that may or may not also be present. Homocysteine is a normal breakdown product of the essential amino acid methionine, which contributes methyl groups to brain neurotransmitters such as serotonin, dopamine, and noradrenaline. It appears that homocysteine works together with high cholesterol, instigating the small endothelial lining ruptures and accelerating the clot formation that can cut off the blood flow.

In addition to the complications of plaque leaking into the coronary artery due to this rupture, the artery also responds to stop the blood from flowing "out of it" by constricting (even though the blood is, in fact, not flowing out of it). If this constriction and the blood clot formation work together to the point of completely stopping the blood from reaching the heart, it can cause death to that part of the heart. A "heart attack," by definition, is when a portion of the heart muscle dies due to a lack of blood flow.

The accepted procedure once a heart

attack has begun is to either use clot-busting drugs or do an emergency angioplasty. The latter is when doctors open the blocked artery by putting a catheter through the middle of the clot, inflating it to break the clot apart, and then placing a stint into it to keep the artery open. That quick procedure usually costs between twenty and thirty thousand dollars!

Of course, these are emergency measures that don't address the root of the problem—the plaque that may be hidden away in the artery wall. The key is to avoid putting the plaque there in the first place, find a way to remove what is already there, or stop the ruptures that allow it to flow into the blood.

Another result of this same process is a stroke. Sixty-one percent of strokes occur in basically the same way, only the blockages occur in the arteries feeding the brain rather than the heart (these are called *thrombotic* or *ischemic* strokes—or are referred to medically as *atherothrombotic brain infarctions*). Atherosclerosis of the carotid arteries (those feeding the brain) is called cerebrovascular or carotid artery disease. This type of stroke is basically a "heart attack in the brain." The other forms of strokes occur because of a clot breaking off from another place in the blood system and lodging in the carotid arteries to cause a blockage, or when a carotid or other vessel feeding the brain bursts because of an aneurysm, causing blood to flow out into a body cavity rather than into the brain. Overall, strokes are the leading cause of serious, long-term disability in the United States today.[4]

Taking on Goliath

Though I have not had room in this chapter to go into all the nuances of all the different forms of cardiovascular disease, I believe this brief summary will help you to understand enough about it to see how the solutions I will discuss in the following chapters address these diseases. I also believe that knowledge helps us to overcome fear. Now that we have taken a good look at the Goliath of heart disease, I trust you know enough to overcome the fear with which our adversary would paralyze us concerning it. It is time to arm ourselves with the weapons that will defeat it.

Chapter 3

THE FIVE SMOOTH STONES THAT WILL DEFEAT CARDIOVASCULAR DISEASE

Chapter 3

THE FIVE SMOOTH STONES THAT WILL DEFEAT CARDIOVASCULAR DISEASE

Before David faced Goliath, he went to a brookside and found five smooth stones (rounded over time by the water). He chose smooth stones because they were perfect for his task. Neither did he wait nor delay until he was older to do this, but he did it in his youth.

No matter how old we are, the time is now to address the Goliath of cardiovascular disease that we all face. If we can confront it in our youth, so much the better, but if we are older, the day to start is still today. The "five smooth stones" for slaying this giant that we will discuss in this chapter are smooth, because it will take most of them a period of time to work. These may well be lifestyle changes for many of us—something that you will start today but never stop doing—while others are things you are already doing and should continue to do. Whereas it only took David one stone to slay his Goliath, we will need to use most, if not all, of these steps to prevent CVD from gaining a foothold in our lives.

Here are the five main things I feel we need to do to prevent—or reverse—the damage of cardiovascular disease:

(1) Stop smoking and avoid second-

hand smoke.

(2) Exercise and control our weight.
(3) Adopt a low-fat, low-cholesterol, low-sodium, high-fiber diet.
(4) Begin a basic daily vitamin and nutritional supplement program.
(5) Use other natural compounds that specifically address cardiovascular disease.

Each of these address, directly or indirectly, one or more of the main causes of cardiovascular disease listed below:

- *Primary Causes/Indicators*
  Cigarette smoke
  Hypertension (high blood pressure)
  High cholesterol, or a high LDL/HDL cholesterol ratio
  High levels of homocysteine

- *Secondary Causes/Indicators*
  Family history
  Being overweight/obese
  Lack of exercise
  Diabetes
  Hyperthyroidism
  High levels of triglycerides
  Stress
  Aging
  Nutritional deficiencies of certain vitamins, minerals, and essential fatty acids

STOP SMOKING AND AVOID SECONDHAND SMOKE

Studies have shown time and again that smoking is one of the major causes of chronic illness, whether it is heart disease, cancer, emphysema, or a number of other problems. Daily exposure to cigarette smoke adversely affects all parts of the cardiovascular system. Nicotine damages the linings of the blood vessels, increases the heart rate, constricts the arteries, and thus hampers the flow of oxygen and other nutrients to all parts of the body as well as increasing the risk of carbon monoxide intoxication. Many toxic minerals are found in cigarette smoke, including cadmium, which raises blood pressure. Smoking also increases bad (LDL and VLDL) cholesterol levels, thus increasing the chances of atherosclerosis, high blood pressure, and their complications. As we have already mentioned, cigarette smoke is also a considerable source of free radicals that do a great deal of damage to our cells and body tissues. These can lead to heart disease, cancer, premature aging, and other complications. Smoking is not only one of the primary indicators of CVD, but it also contributes to two of the others (hypertension and high cholesterol levels). Thus, one of the most effective steps in CVD prevention is to stop smoking.

While I am confident that many of you do not smoke, I would also caution you to be wary of secondhand smoke and other air pollutants. Many studies have shown that secondhand smoke can be even more potent than what a smoker takes in through his or her own habit. If you are in an area or job situation where you are continually exposed to cigarette smoke—which, thank God, are becoming fewer and fewer—you need to start praying about making some immediate changes.

EXERCISE AND CONTROL WEIGHT

Lack of exercise and being overweight or obese are not only risk factors for CVD but also contribute to other risk factors. Lack of exercise over time weakens the heart and other muscles, allows the blood vessel linings to harden, weakens blood flow, and contributes to being overweight, while exercising actually reverses all of these trends. Being overweight, or going on to being obese (by definition, being at least thirty pounds overweight), contributes to both atherosclerosis and high blood pressure because of the increased body fats and poor good (HDL) to bad (LDL & VLDL) cholesterol ratio. It also contributes to diabetes, which is another risk factor for heart disease. By achieving your proper weight through eating the right foods and exercise, you address all of these risk factors at once. Regular exercise has also been shown to help us cope with stress, which is yet another factor in heart disease.

We will discuss diet more in the next section, but when I talk about getting enough exercise, I am referring to something as simple as walking for forty to forty-five minutes, three to five times a week, or taking a brisk walk every day for about twenty minutes. This is enough to get your heart rate up and doesn't require an expensive membership to a health club. Obviously, you could do more (it is advisable to start with less if you find this too challenging), but I have always believed in starting with simple changes and then working your way up as God leads you. It is also important not to start with too much activity, since that can

The Five Smooth Stones

stress your system more than help it.

Walking, jogging, stationary cycling, outdoor cycling, water exercise, tennis, stretching, aerobic exercise, and swimming are all fine workouts. In at least one study, walking alone proved to return elasticity to artery walls. The important thing is to find something you enjoy and can do regularly that exercises and builds the aerobic capacity of your heart, lungs, and other body systems. As you improve your fitness, you can combine various forms of exercise to address all the muscle groups and body systems. Remember to do proper warm-ups and cool-downs. It is also better to eat after exercising rather than before, as exercise contributes to food absorption and burning calories.

DETERMINE YOUR SAFE HEART-RATE RANGE

Whatever exercise you choose, do it vigorously enough to get your heart rate elevated during the time you are exercising. Physical fitness experts have a simple formula for determining a safe heart-rate range for exercising. Simply subtract your age from 220 to find your maximum heart rate. For instance, if you are forty years old, your formula would be 220-40 = 180. Your target heart-rate zone is between 60 and 80 percent of that number. So multiply your maximum heart rate by 0.6 for the bottom of your safe exercise range and by 0.8 for the top. As you exercise, check your pulse rate now and then to be sure your heartbeat is within that range. Using the example above, the safe heart-rate range for a forty-year-old would be 108 to 144.

Find your pulse in your wrist or neck, count the number of heartbeats in ten seconds, and multiply that number by six. If the number you get is within your safe exercise range, you're fine. If it's lower, work harder. If it's higher, slow down a little. When starting an exercise program, aim at the lowest part of your target zone for the first few weeks. Gradually build up to the higher part of your target zone.

ADOPT A LOW-FAT, LOW-CHOLESTEROL, LOW-SODIUM, HIGH-FIBER DIET

If you have read any of my other books (particularly *The Bible Cure*), you will know that I have long been a proponent of what is called the Mediterranean diet. This is a diet that is low in red meats, hydrogenated oils, and processed foods (major sources of bad fats and cholesterols), and high in fiber, nuts, fish, fruits, vegetables (especially salads), and olive oil (sources of good fats and cholesterols and other nutrients our bodies need)—all of which are also mentioned in the Bible and are the staples of dishes from Israel, Greece, Italy, and other nations that surround the Mediterranean Sea.

THE MEDITERRANEAN DIET

If you were to look at their menus, you would see that the following items make up most of what is eaten in the Mediterranean region every day:

(1) *Olive oil*. Olive oil replaces most fats, oils, butter, and margarine, all of which contribute LDL choles-

terol to the diet. On the contrary, olive oil raises the high-density lipoprotein (HDL), or "good" cholesterol, levels and appears to strengthen the immune system. Extra-virgin olive oil is preferred over other varieties.

(2) *Breads.* Dark, chewy, high-fiber, crusty bread is present at most meals in the Mediterranean region. Another good choice is Ezekiel bread, which is a recipe based on Ezekiel 4:9. (Typical American white bread made from processed white flour is not part of this diet.)

(3) *Pasta, rice, couscous, bulgur, potatoes.* Pasta is often served with fresh vegetables and herbs sautéed in olive oil; occasionally it is served with small quantities of lean beef.

Tomato sauces, often served with pasta, are high in lycopene, one of the most potent antioxidants (substances that absorb or salvage harmful free radicals). Dark rice is preferred. Couscous and bulgur are other forms of whole grains.

(4) *Grains.* To obtain healthy grains from many different sources, eat cereals containing wheat bran (one-half cup, four to five times a week), or alternate with cereals such as Bran Buds (one-half cup) or those containing oat bran (one-third cup)—all of which contain water-soluble fibers that lower cholesterol. Bran Buds in particular is a great CVD fighter because it contains psyllium, a water-soluble fiber that can reduce the risk of

CVD by 15 percent if eaten twice daily. Psyllium lowers both overall cholesterol levels and especially LDL cholesterol levels. Eating this with soy milk rather than regular milk adds extra benefits because soy is a whole protein and also further reduces cholesterol (for more information on soy, see the next subsection).

(5) *Fruits.* Several different fruits are available in the Mediterranean region, and they are usually eaten raw and at least two or three times a day. Bananas in particular are not only high in potassium, which has been shown in studies to lower blood pressure, but also appear to have natural ACE inhibitors. (ACE inhibitors are one of the

most popular classes of drugs prescribed to treat heart disease and have almost no side effects.) Studies have shown that two bananas a day can lower blood pressure up to 10 percent.

(6) *Beans.* Various kinds of beans should be included in your diet: pinto, great northern, navy, lentils, kidney beans, etc. Bean and lentil soups are very popular in the Mediterranean countries and are usually prepared with a small amount of olive oil. You should have about one-half cup of beans three or four times a week.

(7) *Nuts.* Ten unsalted almonds or walnuts a day have some incredible benefits. Almonds, in particular, are higher in dietary fiber than

most other nuts, and the fiber in almonds seems uniquely effective in lowering overall cholesterol levels, better even than olive oil. They also contain plant sterols as well as saponins and the protein arginine (which we will discuss more in chapter 5), all of which lower the risk of heart disease. Various research studies have reported that consuming almonds and such nuts regularly can reduce the risk of heart disease by 35 to 57 percent.

(8) *Vegetables and herbs.* Dark green vegetables are prominent in the Mediterranean diet, especially in salads. The updated food pyramid that has recently been appearing in science and news magazines suggests that vegetables should be

eaten daily "in abundance." I suggest that you eat at least one of the following cruciferous vegetables daily: cabbage, broccoli, cauliflower, turnip greens, or mustard greens; and at least one from the following group of fruits and vegetables daily: carrots, spinach, sweet potatoes, cantaloupe, peaches, or apricots. Raw onions have been shown to raise good (HDL) cholesterol levels, while more and more studies are showing that the equivalent of one clove of garlic a day (used widely in the Mediterranean) can protect against free radicals, reduce blood pressure, counter the tendency of blood to clot, as well as lower overall cholesterol levels.

(9) *Yogurt.* Eating fat-free, live-culture yogurt daily has some incredible benefits as well. The live bacteria in yogurt (lactobacillus, streptococcus, and acidophilus) significantly strengthen the immune system, which is good for all our other body systems as well as the cardiovascular system (freezing yogurt, as is often done to make a dessert, kills these good bacteria). A light breakfast of one cup of fat-free yogurt with ten almonds and chopped fruit sprinkled on it is a great start to the day. Since most heart attacks and strokes tend to occur between six o'clock in the morning and noon (peaking between eight and ten o'clock), a light breakfast such as this goes a

long way in reducing the platelet stickiness that contributes to the clotting that causes heart attacks. Eating yogurt with your morning nutritional supplements also reduces the "vitamin taste" that can often linger after taking tablets and capsules alone. Another low-fat breakfast alternative would be oatmeal or Bran Flakes with soy milk (or low-fat milk) and fruit and six ounces of Concord grape or orange juice. Either of these is a heart-healthy alternative to the more traditional high-cholesterol American breakfast of sausages, eggs, pancakes, French toast, and/or sugary cereals with whole milk.

(10) *Cheeses.* Mediterranean countries tend to eat lighter-colored or

white dairy or goat cheeses, usually grated or broken up on salads or in small wedges combined with fruit for a dessert. Unlike other milk products, recent studies indicate that cheese might not contribute to clogged arteries as much as was previously believed. Still, it is wise to eat reduced- or low-fat cheeses (fat-free cheeses are often rubbery and not very palatable).

While all of these should be eaten daily, red meat, fish, poultry, and eggs, on the other hand, should be eaten only a few times a week. I would put these in the following order of frequency and importance:

(1) *Fish*. Cold-water fish high in omega–3 fatty acids, such as cod,

salmon, mackerel, and herring are best; trout is also good. Because of the benefits of these essential fatty acids for our cardiovascular system, the American Heart Association has recently advised those who have had a coronary heart disease event to take a daily supplement of one ounce of "fish oils" every day.[1] Fish is the healthiest meat we can have in our diet.

(2) *Poultry*. White breast meat without the skin is best. Poultry can be eaten two or three times a week.

(3) *Eggs*. Eggs should be eaten no more than two or three times a week.

(4) *Red meat*. The fat in red meat is the worst fat we can consume. When God commanded His peo-

ple to avoid fat in Leviticus 3:17 and 7:23, I believe this is the type of fat He was referring to. The fat and cholesterol from red meat are the main contributors to the fatty plaques that can plug our arteries or create the sudden blockages that cause heart attacks or strokes. Red meat eaten in Mediterranean countries tends to be much leaner and is eaten only two or three times a month. If you do include red meat in a meal, be sure to eat small portions of lean meat and trim whatever fat you can before you cook it.

While the Mediterranean diet is not an absolute for heart health, it does give us a great guideline for how and what we should eat to keep our cardiovascular and other systems healthy. While changing our diet is probably one of the more difficult on this list of five things to do, it is also one of the most beneficial. Switching from the typical American diet of processed and fatty red meats and starchy foods to one made up of salads, soups, whole grains, fruits and vegetables, and olive or canola oil is not only one of the healthiest things you can do, but it could also prove to make the difference between being satisfied with long life (see Psalm 91:16) and suffering a sudden death at the hands of the Goliath of cardiovascular disease.

SOYBEANS: THE PLANT KINGDOM'S BEST PROTEIN SUBSTITUTE

While the soybean is not necessarily a part of the Mediterranean diet, it has several beneficial characteristics that make it worth mentioning here. First of all, it is an excellent protein substitute for red meat. You can receive whole proteins from the plant kingdom by combining certain vegetables (beans and rice or corn, for example), but soy is the only plant that is a complete protein in and of itself. In other words, it is the only plant that has all the essential amino acids necessary for the formation of proteins in one package.

Soy also contains isoflavones, which are flavonoids (also often called bioflavonoids), a major category of plant antioxidants. These isoflavones appear to slow the oxidation of LDL cholesterol, which is the process that turns it into the fatty plaques that can lodge themselves in the walls of our blood vessels. They also inhibit the production of adhesive proteins and other factors that trigger the binding of certain immune cells to the artery walls, a first step in inflammation and damage to the interior lining of the vessels. Isoflavones also appear to help dilate the vessels, which will keep the blood flowing smoothly.

Soy is now available in a variety of products from tofu to tempeh, soy ice cream, milk, yogurt, cheese, flour, and even roasted soy nuts. Tofu is perhaps the most popular form. It has no real flavor of its own but absorbs flavor from whatever it is cooked with. It can easily be worked into a wide variety of recipes and tastes. To be honest, my wife, Linda, and I have never been able to work tofu into our diets because the texture seems so odd to us. Of course, we encourage you to at least try it, but we can definitely understand if you choose another way to get the benefits of soy!

The way we have worked around this is to drink soy milk. We regularly have soy milk on our breakfast cereal (we started with vanilla soy milk) and have found a variety of others that we like, including chocolate and "creamy" (this is not mixed with cream, but is thickened with other natural proteins).

Soy has other tremendous cardiovascular system benefits besides its ability to replace red meat as a source of protein. The FDA has even given soy product packagers the freedom to print on their labels that soy may reduce heart disease, because it lowers both total and LDL cholesterol levels and reduces the chance of blood clot formation.

Addressing Cholesterol Specifically

You have probably picked up a major trend in all we have discussed so far that is also worth addressing more directly: that is, the need to reduce overall cholesterol levels and improve the ratio of good (HDL) to bad (LDL and VLDL) cholesterol in our system. For reference sake, HDL refers to "high-density lipoprotein" cholesterol, while LDL and VLDL refer to "low-density lipoprotein" or "very low-density lipoprotein" cholesterols. As a whole, cholesterols are easy to absorb and hard to eliminate. They are all fat-protein molecules that carry non-immersible fats through the blood. HDL cholesterol is considered "good" because it carries these non-immersible fats out of the blood and to the liver, where they can be "cleaned up," and thus reduces the overall levels of cholesterol in the blood; LDL carries them to the cells and usually makes up most of the cholesterol in the blood; while VLDL cholesterol appears to merely keep these fats in circulation and may be the greatest risk for the development of atherosclerosis.

This is why eating high-fiber foods and other things that absorb cholesterol and take it out of the system is a good practice, as well as minimizing cholesterol intake in the first place—especially LDL and VLDL cholesterols. The general suggested maximum for cholesterol intake is 300 milligrams daily—about the amount of cholesterol in one egg yolk (275 milligrams). If you are at risk for CVD because of family heredity or signs of it having been found during a regular checkup, it is a good idea to consume no more than 150 milligrams of cholesterol a day. This is why there has been such a big push for more vegetarian diets.

Thus, the goal of addressing cholesterol in our diet is to lower overall cholesterol, but more important, to lower LDL and VLDL cholesterols in ratio to HDL cholesterol, which, as we have said, helps fight the bad cholesterols. As a rule of thumb, saturated fats (butter, milk, red meats, margarines, poultry, avocados, etc.) are more likely to develop bad cholesterols, while monounsaturated fats (olive oil, canola oil, almonds, walnuts, fish, etc.) tend to have a neutral effect on cholesterol levels or slightly favor HDLs over LDLs; polyunsaturated fats (oils from sesame, safflower, corn, soybeans, and other such sources) tend to lower both good and bad cholesterol levels. Statistical studies of the relationship between cholesterol consumption and the risk of CVD have suggested that for every 1 percent drop in cholesterol, the risks of CVD drop 2 to 3 percent. This is why paying particular attention to this one CVD cause can be so important in preventing the problems and complications associated with it.

High Cholesterol May Be a Result of Low Thyroid Output

After a diet that is high in saturated fats, the second leading cause of elevated cholesterol is a low output from the thyroid gland. Even mild hypothyroidism can significantly raise the potential risk of heart disease. This is because a low output from the thyroid gland slows the body's ability to break down and metabolize cholesterol, thus raising its level in the bloodstream. Some 13 million Americans have low thyroid output, and half of them do not know it.

This is why I suggest that you ask your doctor about taking a simple TSH blood test during your regular checkups, especially if you show high blood cholesterol or have a concern about it. If it should turn out that you do have some form of hypothyroidism, it is easily treated with Armour thyroid or levothyroxine, which your doctor can prescribe for you as needed.

Begin a Basic Daily Vitamin and Nutritional Supplement Program

While eating right is a major key to preventing CVD, it is important to also remember that because of modern, mass-production farming techniques, the nutritional value of our foods is not what it used to be. While the traditional view of the medical community was that we can get all the nutrients our bodies need daily from what we eat, now the medical community is beginning to endorse taking daily vitamin supplements, because they have been shown to be so effective in preventing chronic illnesses such as cardiovascular disease.[2] The American Heart Association is suggesting that those who have had coronary heart disease events (such as chest pains or a heart attack) should take essential fatty acid capsules daily.[3] God has given us incredible abilities to put the nutrients we are lacking into extracts to supplement our diet, which may be the extra edge we need to keep sickness from our midst. (See Exodus 23:25–26.)

God's Pathway to Healing: HEART

With so many studies showing the benefits of nutritional supplements and the general suboptimal level of these nutrients in our food, I firmly endorse that everyone begin a daily basic nutritional supplement program. If you are not especially concerned about cardiovascular disease or other chronic sickness, taking daily supplements may be the key to keeping you from ever having to worry about them. A good program will not only include vitamins and minerals but also fruit, vegetable, and herbal extracts; enzymes for absorption and digestion; marine oils; flavonoids; and other key nutrients. (For a complete list of recommended compounds for a good daily nutritional supplement program, see my pocket book *God's Pathway to Healing: Vitamins and Supplements,* or visit our Web site: *www.abundantnutrition.com.*)

Use Other Natural Compounds That Specifically Address Cardiovascular Disease

While our heart and blood vessels can definitely benefit from a basic daily nutritional supplement program, there are also certain natural compounds you can take if you are specifically concerned about heart arrhythmias, hypertension (high blood pressure), or cardiovascular disease in general because of heredity, warning signs, or if you have suffered a coronary heart disease event. These would be taken in addition to your basic nutritional support program. Please check with your family physician for proper dosages and to see which of these will benefit you the most for your specific pathway to healing. It is important to remember, though, that many of these compounds work best when taken together, so make sure you not only take the right ones but also take them in the right combinations.

Natural Compounds to Address Cardiovascular Disease in General

L-ARGININE. L-arginine (often referred to simply as "arginine") is an amino acid that is a precursor of nitric oxide. Nitric oxide, produced in the body, increases blood flow in the coronary arteries because it dilates blood vessels and inhibits blood clot formation by decreasing the stickiness of platelets. It also stops the reflex artery spasms that can occur if the lining of a blood vessel ruptures and thus helps it through this acute and dangerous period without the spasms further cutting off blood flow. It is considered a tremendous circulation enhancer.

Our blood vessels can constrict for up to six to eight hours after large, fatty meals (something we should avoid), which is why so many heart attacks occur after such meals. If you have high levels of arginine in your bloodstream, however, it can counter this constriction and keep the blood flowing smoothly despite the fact that there may be some significant plaque buildup in the arteries.

ASPIRIN. Various studies suggest that taking low-dose aspirin (81 milligrams) can prevent one out of three heart attacks. Aspirin acts as a natural blood thinner and thus improves circulation. However, those who are allergic to aspirin or are already on a blood-thinning medication should avoid aspirin. Personally, I take 81 milligrams of aspirin daily along with my other nutritional supplements. This is something you should pray about and ask your doctor about, particularly if there is a history of elevated cholesterol or cardiovascular disease in your family.

B-VITAMINS AND BETAINE. Studies indicate that folate (folic acid), B_6, and B_{12} all reduce homocysteine levels in the blood. According to some experts, folate supplements could reduce the number of heart disease deaths by 50,000 every year [4] (at the present time, roughly 946,000 die each year from cardiovascular disease).[5] Since high homocysteine levels lead to twice the risk for heart disease as low homocysteine levels, taking these three B-vitamins regularly could cut your risks of CVD in half. Betaine (trimethylglycine), a dietary supplement, also works with the B-vitamins to lower dangerous homocysteine levels.

COENZYME Q10 (UBIQUINONE). CoQ10 is a pigment found in plants, chlorophyll or lycopene. It is involved in the manufacture of adenosine triphosphate (ATP), which is the basic fuel that creates energy for the cells of the body. CoQ10 seems to especially benefit the cells of the heart muscle and is one of the only substances that strengthens heart contractions. It also helps stabilize the electrical activity of the heart, which gives the impulses that regulate the heartbeat. Patients who have suffered heart attacks, congestive heart failure, cardiomyopathy (any condition that damages and weakens the heart muscle), and irregular heartbeats have shown to be deficient in CoQ10. Those taking CoQ10 after heart surgery recuperated more rapidly and had fewer problems. It also seems to act as an antioxidant to combat free radicals.

One downside of many cholesterol-lowering statin drugs, such as Zocor, Pravachol, Lipitor, and Mevacor, taken to help prevent heart disease, is that they appear to interfere with the production of CoQ10. Some antihypertensive drugs have the same effect. However, daily supplements of this valuable nutrient can easily compensate for this.

DOCOSAHEXAENOIC ACID (DHA) AND EICOSAPENTAENOIC ACID (EPA). These omega-3 fatty acids are the most beneficial found in cold-water fish, such as cod, herring, mackerel, and salmon; dark leafy vegetables; grains, seeds, and nuts; or in marine oil supplements. There is a range of possibilities for how these benefit the cardiovascular system, among which are the reduction of blood lipids and the production of thromboxane A_2, which is one of the agents that activates platelet clumping or clotting. They also appear to reduce the risk of ventricular fibrillation (a rapid arrhythmia of the ventricles, which prevents them from pumping blood effectively and can lead quickly to death—this often happens prior to cardiac arrest, which is when the heart simply stops beating) and decrease blood pressure. A double-blind test showed that people with atherosclerosis who took fish oil capsules regularly for two years had a significant regression of atherosclerotic plaques and a decrease in cardiovascular disease events over those who did not.[6]

GARLIC BULB EXTRACT. Garlic has numerous phytochemicals that help normalize blood pressure, reduce platelet stickiness, regulate blood lipid levels, and reduce atherosclerotic plaque formation.

GREEN TEA EXTRACT. This extract is a natural source of catechin antioxidants and polyphenols, which help prevent LDL cholesterol from oxidizing—the process causes it to be deposited in the walls of the blood vessels. It also helps to dilate blood vessels to improve blood flow. The flavonoids in green tea stop inflammation in the arteries and relax them, both of which work to keep these blood vessels elastic and responsive to the pulsing of the blood flowing through them, further improving circulation. All of this is extremely important for getting blood to our peripheral body tissues, particularly our hands and feet. Cold hands and feet can indicate that we are not getting enough circulation to these areas.

To get the same results as the extract, you would have to drink three or four cups of green tea a day, which is possible but not always convenient. This is why taking this in a supplement form is easier to do more consistently and thus is more beneficial.

GRAPE-SEED AND GRAPE-SKIN EXTRACTS. These extracts are natural sources of anthocyanidin antioxidants, which reduce blood clotting. Grape-skin extract also contains the antioxidant *resveratrol*, which decreases blood platelet stickiness and helps keep blood vessels open and flexible. This is also the compound that may be the answer to what is called "The French Paradox"—the French diet is high in cream, butter, meat, and other saturated fats but causes relatively low levels of heart disease. Many experts say this is because of the resveratrol that is in the red wine that the French drink with most of their meals. I, however, have always endorsed getting it through extracts or non-alcoholic red wine because of the negative effects alcohol can have on the system.

Grape-seed extract has the uncommon ability to raise HDL cholesterol levels up to 14 percent (niacin also does this but has some unpleasant side effects, such as flushing and dizziness). Studies indicate that for every 1 percent increase in HDL cholesterol, there is a 3 percent drop in risk of heart attack. It also appears to drop triglyceride levels (another significant factor in causing cardiovascular disease) by as much as 15 percent. It appears that grape-seed extract from red grapes has significantly more powerful antioxidants than the well-known antioxidants vitamin C, vitamin E, and beta carotene.

HAWTHORN. This herb extract that comes from the hawthorn plant (a member of the rose family) has a direct effect on the electrical activity and conduction in the heart muscle and thus strengthens the heart, regulates heart rhythm, and helps normalize blood pressure. It also inhibits blood clot formation and decreases cholesterol levels. Its use to treat heart disease dates back to Roman times, because it had been found effective in treating dropsy (called congestive heart disease today). It is a rich source of flavonoids and pycnogenols—plant-derived antioxidants—and phytochemicals, such as saponins.

While it has not been shown as effective for treating coronary heart failure as the

ACE inhibitors in many studies, it does work well to supplement the effects of the ACE drugs. Also remember that many of these compounds work best together, and most research is done using only one compound at a time to limit variables. If you are using these natural supplements regularly, you may soon find your doctor reducing your prescribed dosage of ACE inhibitors or even taking you off of them altogether. Hawthorn alone, however, has been proven to be significantly effective in treating angina (chest pains) and minor arrhythmias (or "heart palpitations").

MAGNESIUM. This mineral is valuable for energy metabolism in the heart (thus helping to regulate the heartbeat) and appears to work with calcium and potassium to regulate blood pressure. It has also been called "nature's calcium channel blocker" because it blocks calcium from entering into muscle and heart tissue, making them less elastic. There is also some evidence to suggest that magnesium protects against the atherosclerotic effects of hydrogenated oils (margarine-like fats found in many junk foods). Magnesium is also one of the few essential nutrients for which deficiencies are very common, therefore one to which we also need to pay special attention.

NOTOGINSENG. This herb (also called pseudoginseng or panax pseudoginseng), from the notoginseng root, improves blood flow and helps regulate heart rhythm by helping to stabilize the electrical activity of the heart.

POLICOSANOL. This extract from the waxy

discarded by-product of sugar cane during sugar production is being shown again and again as an effective balancer of cholesterol levels, and it reduces inflammation in the artery lining. It is easily one of the most significant breakthroughs in the natural treatment of heart disease because it can go head to head with the statin drugs we discussed a bit earlier but does not have the side effects of muscle aches and pains or liver problems. (Those on statin drugs have to have regular liver enzyme checks. The only "adverse" side effect of policosanol, it appears, is that sometimes those taking it lose a few pounds, if you can call that adverse!) It also seems more effective than statin drugs in some surprising ways. While both policosanol and the statin drugs can lower LDL cholesterol levels by up to 20 percent, policosanol can raise HDL cholesterol levels an average of 13 to 15 percent, which is better than the statin drugs. It also has been proven to inhibit the formation of lesions in the arteries, keep LDL cholesterol from oxidizing, increase exercise endurance, reduce the manufacture of thromboxane A10 (an inflammation promoter), and reduces platelet stickiness. It is also much less expensive than the statin drugs and is now increasingly being considered to replace them.

The greatest benefit of lowering the ratio of LDL to HDL in the cardiovascular system, in conjunction with strengthening the heart's contractions and dilating the vessels, is that it accelerates HDL's ability to *remove* bad cholesterol from the artery and vein walls. All of these God-given substances working together can then *reverse* atherosclerosis and the other cardiovascular diseases to which it often leads—something many doctors did not believe possible less than a decade ago.

TAURINE. This amino acid has a direct effect on calming and stabilizing the electrical conduction in the heart muscle, thus helping to regulate heart rhythm. It has been proven to have a significant positive effect in treating congestive heart failure (even more effective than CoQ10 in at least one study).[7]

TOCOTRIENOLS. These are the cousins of the vitamin E tocopherols. These are important antioxidants and also help regulate cholesterol and may prevent LDL cholesterol from oxidizing, thus also reducing atherosclerotic plaques. The tocotrienols work very effectively when combined with policosanol.

CARDIOVASCULAR DISEASE CAN BE BEATEN

Because of the awareness focused on cardiovascular disease, death rates due to it have actually declined in the last decade. By combining the five "stones" in this list, the same can happen for you. God's guidelines for healthy eating, exercise, and the compounds God provided for our health in His natural creation are all signposts on the way to the fulfillment of His promises. As we walk on His pathway to healing cardiovascular disease, we must heed them in order to achieve their desired end—a long and satisfying, full life. (See Psalm 91:16; Proverbs 9:11; John 10:10.)

Chapter 4

SPECIFICALLY COMBATING HYPERTENSION AND HEART ARRHYTHMIA

Chapter 4

SPECIFICALLY COMBATING HYPERTENSION AND HEART ARRHYTHMIA

While all of the steps in the previous chapter will go a long way in battling all forms of cardiovascular disease, I want to make some specific comments here about two of the most dangerous: hypertension (high blood pressure) and heart arrhythmia (irregular heartbeats or heart palpitations). While hypertension is a key cause of both heart attacks and strokes, heart arrhythmia (though quite common in all of us) can be the culminating event before cardiac arrest (when the heart suddenly stops beating). Both of these are key reasons why regular checkups are vital to our continuing health and well-being.

Natural Compounds to Combat Hypertension

Hypertension (high blood pressure) is the most pervasive of all major cardiovascular heart diseases, affecting roughly 50 million Americans (the next most common—which is coronary heart disease—affects just over one quarter of the same number at 12.9 million).[1] It is called the "silent killer" because it has few symptoms other than a blood pressure reading to indicate its presence before it erupts into something fatal. By definition, a person who has hypertension is (1) anyone with a blood pressure reading of 140/90 or higher, or (2) anyone who is on antihypertensive medications. However, God has provided some helpful natural compounds to help us on our pathway to healing hypertension, and many have been shown to be effective in either reducing the dosages of antihypertensive meds or eliminating the need for them completely.

Of course, all of the steps in the preceding chapter apply to treating hypertension, but I would also like to make special mention of three here that should be most carefully considered if you are battling it:

(1) *Potassium*. At least thirty-three different studies I have seen show that

potassium (of which bananas are a great source, though it is also available in supplement form) can reduce blood pressure. I normally recommend taking 99 milligrams of potassium in the citrate form on a daily basis, and then any additional potassium that you get from your food simply builds on this.

(2) *Polyphenols*. An article in the medical journal *Archives of Internal Medicine* stated that two tablespoons of cold-pressed, extra-virgin olive oil (a good source of polyphenols) taken every day over a period of time resulted in a marked reduction in the required dosage of blood pressure medications. In fact, many were able to cut their prescriptions in half after only a few

months, while a quarter of them were able to control their blood pressure without any prescriptions at all.[2] This is believed to be the result of the polyphenols stimulating the production of nitric oxide (which causes blood vessels to dilate and relax) and their antioxidant activities.

(3) *Magnesium.* The "Honolulu Heart Study" showed that magnesium was the substance that showed the strongest correlation with lowering both systolic (the high point when the heart beats) and diastolic (the low point when the heart rests) blood pressures.[3] Low magnesium levels correlate strongly with the hardening and clogging of the arteries in atherosclerosis, both of

which greatly contribute to high blood pressure. While magnesium deficiency has increased in recent decades, hypertension has also risen in epidemic proportions. (For more on the benefits of magnesium, see the previous chapter.)

Natural Compounds to Combat Heart Arrhythmia

Studies have shown that all of us have occasional irregular heartbeats (also referred to as palpitations), though most of the time we are not even aware of it. Some notice irregular heartbeats throughout the day, while others notice them when they are quiet and particularly when they lie down to sleep at night. Personally, I notice them from time to time when I lie down, especially if I have eaten a large meal late in the evening (something I don't do very often). A slowed heartbeat combined with the diversion of blood into the digestive tract to help absorb the nutrients from the food often contribute to these minor and benign irregularities. However, as an irregular heartbeat is also the culminating event that precedes cardiac arrest, it is something we should get checked out and do what we can to prevent.

The most common type of heart arrhythmia (irregular heartbeats) is really premature contractions of the large pumping chamber of the heart. After a premature beat, there is a slightly longer pause in the heart rate, which we sometimes call a "skipped heartbeat." It is usually this longer pause that gets our attention.

Of the compounds that we have

God's Pathway to Healing: HEART

discussed in detail in the previous chapter, there are five that generally help control this premature beat pattern and assist in leveling out and controlling our heart rhythms. In this list, I have included in parentheses the daily dosages of each that I recommend to specifically treat heart arrhythmia. Please note that these are total dosages of what you would take every day and are not added to what you may already be receiving from your basic supplement plan: So, for example, if you are already getting 25 milligrams of CoQ10 from your daily supplement, simply add 25 milligrams more to address heartbeat irregularities, not an additional 50 milligrams.

(1) Coenzyme Q10 (50 milligrams)
(2) Hawthorne (250 milligrams)

(3) Magnesium (550 milligrams)
(4) Notoginseng (250 milligrams)
(5) Taurine (400 milligrams)

God Designed These Compounds to Work Together

In taking any supplements, remember this important principle: They work best in combination. A smaller amount of a couple of different compounds often works more effectively than a much larger dose of any one. They have a synergistic effect. This is a pattern we see in God's plant kingdom. God did not put only one nutrient into one plant, nor did He expect us to eat only one food alone at a meal or the same foods at every meal. This is because there are various nutrients that work together to give us the nutrition we need. Remember this pattern when you are supplementing your diet to address health concerns as you seek God's pathway to healing.

Chapter 5

YOUR DAILY WALK ON THE PATHWAY TO A HEALTHY HEART AND CARDIOVASCULAR SYSTEM

Chapter 5

YOUR DAILY WALK ON THE PATHWAY TO A HEALTHY HEART AND CARDIOVASCULAR SYSTEM

"David chose five smooth stones out of the brook ... and prevailed over Goliath with a sling and with a stone, and smote the giant, and slew him" (1 Samuel 17:40, 50, paraphrased).

As God led David to victory over Goliath, I believe He will also lead those of us who are willing and obedient to a similar victory over the giant of heart disease. Just hearing the truth is not enough—you have to act on the truths you have heard. Take the following steps to make sure you activate God's unique plan for a healthy heart and cardiovascular system for you.

Step 1: Consult with a physician or reliable medical professional. Make sure you have regular checkups to catch potential problems early, when they are easiest to treat and correct. Many say they don't need to go to doctors because they are doing all the things they need to do in order to maintain their health. I believe this can be fear speaking more than wisdom. Having regular checkups not only keeps you from unnecessary worry about your health but also gives you an opportunity to discuss various cardiovascular disease-defeating strategies with your health professional.

Consultation with a physician or a competent medical professional can give you vital information about your cardiovascular system. As I have said before, these checkups may be the only opportunity to detect conditions such as high blood pressure or an irregular heartbeat because these are normally "silent"—without symptoms. Make sure you discuss with your health advisor all the supplements you may be taking to ensure that there are no conflicts. This person may even be able to suggest packaged supplement programs that contain all or most of what you need to take on a daily basis, making nutritional supplementation even easier. You should also discuss your diet and exercise programs with your doctor to see if he or she has any other advice that might be helpful to you in these areas.

Step 2: Pray with understanding. Seek God in prayer and ask Him to reveal to you and to your doctor the best steps in the natural that you can take to proceed down your pathway to maintaining your health or receiving your healing.

While much of the advice I have offered in this pocket book is practical, do not neglect your daily spiritual needs. Make sure to supplement what you take into your mind and body every day with solid doses of God's Word and prayer. Only then can God lead you into the fullness and abundance of life He has promised you in every area.

If you are not sure how to pray, you can begin by praying a prayer like the following one. Because atherosclerosis is the most

Your Daily Walk on the Pathway...

common foothold for all cardiovascular disease, I have specifically addressed it; from there you can allow God to lead you into praying for your specific health concerns or those of your loved ones:

Father, I thank you in the name of Jesus that my arteries will remain open, my blood flow will remain normal, and my artery walls will not thicken or stiffen. I thank you, Father, that "the life of the flesh is in the blood," according to Leviticus 17:11, and that life will continue to flow to every cell in my body. I thank you that bad cholesterol will not deposit itself in my artery walls and that my cholesterol levels will be normal. I thank you that blood clots will not form on my artery walls, blocking the flow of life through my vessels. Father, I thank you for giving me wisdom to do what I can do to protect this temple from artery blockage and hardening of the arteries.

Allow me to know whether or not I should be on low-dose aspirin to prevent inflammation and blood clots. Guide me to how I should supplement my diet with vitamins and nutritional extracts to give me what I need to keep sickness far from me. I also thank you for guiding me in which medications to take, if any, to lower my cholesterol as part of my pathway to healing. I will be obedient to the guiding of your Holy Spirit. I know that if the Holy Spirit gives me this instruction and direction, I will suffer no side effects from the medications.

Thank you, Father, for setting me free from the generational curse of atherosclerosis and that I will fulfill the number of

*my days according to your promises.
In Jesus' name, I pray. Amen.*

Step 3: Ask the Holy Spirit to guide you into all truth. We have given you a great deal of information about things you can do or take to help your physical body, and it is quite possible that your medical advisor will give you some other options. By referring to the information in this book, you can bring up the discussion of what would be best for you. Ask your health professional if he or she would be willing to work with you in developing a nutritional supplement program or suggest other steps for you to take to combat heart disease.

I strongly encourage you to explore all the aspects of cardiovascular disease that I have shared with you in this book—the pathways that God has created to strengthen and guard your heart, blood, and blood vessels. Pray in faith that God will give you the wisdom you need in order to discern the pathway He has provided that is best for you. It is good to know that in James 1:5 we have God's promise about receiving this wisdom: "If any of you lack wisdom, let him ask of God, that giveth to all men liberally, and upbraideth not; and it shall be given him." Allow the Holy Spirit to guide you into all truth.

Step 4: Maintain proper and healthy nutrition. Exercise your body and mind to stay fit. In other words, dedicate yourself to living the five steps I have outlined for you to defeat cardiovascular disease. Make them a regular part of your lifestyle and remember to make them fun and not a burden. Find a variety of foods and recipes that you like that are part of the Mediterranean diet and experiment with these healthy natural ingredients to create your own delicious meals. Find a means of exercise you enjoy—while some may enjoy walking on a treadmill while watching television, others will need to get outside or find a competitive sport to challenge them or a group to encourage them socially as well. Don't let it become a drudgery, or you won't keep it up over time. Studies have shown that we also need to challenge ourselves intellectually to maintain healthier mental faculties. Establish an active life for an active body and mind.

Step 5: Stand firm in God's pathway to healing for you. Refuse to be discouraged or defeated. Be aggressive in prayer and in faith, claiming your health and healing in Jesus Christ.

GOD HAS A UNIQUE PATHWAY TO CARDIOVASCULAR HEALTH FOR YOU

There are nineteen individually recorded healings in the Gospels, and each is unique in its own way. I believe these are recorded in the Scriptures to show us that God uses different pathways to manifest His healing power. When I realized this, it totally changed the way I practiced medicine. It is incredible to me that when I started praying and asking God to show me, as a doctor, His pathway to healing for each of my patients, I began to see more and more clearly His design for helping each person. Through prayer, faith, knowledge, and wisdom, God can show you His pathway to maintaining health or receiving healing.

If we are simply open to this, God will work miracles. It may be instantaneous, or it may be a process or treatment that takes some time. Just as cardiovascular disease takes some time to develop, it will also take time to reverse it. It may involve certain medicines or even surgery. It may also be a pathway that is relatively uneventful as we remain healthy and have regular checkups. Thank God that we can pray for our healing, but also that we can take precautions before we are sick to avoid the need for healing. Either way, we have tremendous hope.

Hebrews 11:1 says that faith gives substance to those things hoped for. If you don't have anything to hope for, how will faith give substance to it? You have to have hope,

God's Pathway to Healing: HEART

and that hope comes when you know that God has a pathway to health or healing for you. That is a promise you can latch on to, pray for, and have faith in. Thank God for His promises!

These are principles to be applied in all areas of your life, including your physical health. Seek God for answers in the specific areas about which you have concerns. Also see your physician to obtain specific information so you know how to pray. God knows your particular needs and the best way for you to receive your healing and maintain your health. Hang on to the hope of His promises, and He will show you His plan for healthy living that is especially designed for you.

ENDNOTES

Chapter 1

1. "Heart Disease and Stroke Statistics—2003 update," American Heart Association, 17.

Chapter 2

1. Elson M. Haas, M.D., "Nutritional Program for Cardiovascular Disease Prevention," Health World Online: *www.healthy.net/asp/templates/article.asp?PageType@rticle&ID 917.* Accessed: 18 March 2003, excerpted from Elson M. Haas, M.D., *Staying Healthy With Nutrition: The Complete Guide to Diet and Nutritional Medicine* (Berkeley, Calif.: Celestial Arts, 1992).

2. Betsy Bates, "Most Atheromas Lurk in Adventitia, Missed by Angiograms."
3. Stephen R. Daniels, M.D., Ph.D.; Ronald M. Lauer, M.D., et al., "Journal Report 03/06/2003," American Heart Association Online: *www.americanheart.org/presenter.jhtml?identifier 009699.* Accessed: 20 March 2003.
4. "Heart Disease and Stroke Statistics—2003 update" (American Heart Association), 17.

Chapter 3

1. Mitchel L. Zoler, "AHA Endorses Fish Oil Supplements" (15 January 2003): 1, 5.
2. Robert H. Fletcherm, M.D., MSc; and Kathleen M. Farfield, M.D., Ph.D., "Vitamins for Chronic Disease Prevention in Adults: Clinical Applications," *The Journal of the American Medical Association* 287, no. 23 (19 June 2002): 3129.
3. Zoler, "AHA Endorses Fish Oil Supplements."

4. The Natural Pharmacist, "Folate," online at: *www.tnp.com/substance.asp?ID 29.* Accessed: 24 May 2001.

5. American Heart Association, "Heart Disease and Stroke Statistics—2003 update," 5.

6. C. von Schacky, P. Angerer, W. Kothny, et al., "The Effect of Dietary Omega-3 Fatty Acids on Coronary Atherosclerosis: A Randomized, Double-Blind, Placebo-Controlled Trial," *Annals of Internal Medicine* 130 (1999): 554–62.

7. J. Amaza, A. Sawamura, and N. Awata, "Usefulness of Taurine in Chronic Congestive Heart Failure and Its Prospective Application," *Japanese Circulation Journal* 56 (1996): 95–99.

Chapter 4

1. American Heart Association, "Heart Disease and Stroke Statistics—2003 Update," 5.

2. *Archives of Internal Medicine.*

3. "Honolulu Heart Study."

REGINALD B. CHERRY, M.D.—A MEDICAL DOCTOR'S TESTIMONY

The first six years of my life were lived in the dusty rural town of Mansfield, in the Ouachita Mountains of western Arkansas. In those childhood years, I had one seemingly impossible dream—to become a doctor!

Through God's grace, I attended and graduated from Baylor University and the University of Texas Medical School. Throughout those years, I felt God tug on my heart a number of times, especially through Billy Graham as I heard him preach on television. But I never surrendered my life to Jesus Christ.

In my early days of practicing medicine, I met Dr. Kenneth Cooper and became trained in the field of preventive medicine. In the mid-seventies I moved to Houston and established a medical practice for preventive medicine. Unfortunately, at that time money became a driving force in my life.

Nevertheless, God was good to me. He brought into our clinic a nurse who became a Spirit-filled Christian, and she began praying for me. In fact, she had her whole church praying for me!

In my search for fulfillment and meaning in life, I called out to God one night in late November 1979 and prayed, "Jesus, I give you everything I own. I'm sorry for the life

I've lived. I want to live for you the rest of my days. I give you my life." A doctor had been born again. And by the way, that beautiful nurse, Linda, who had prayed for me and shared Jesus with me, is now my wife!

Not only did Jesus transform my life, but He also transformed my medical practice. God spoke to me and said, "I want you to establish a Christian clinic. From now on when you practice medicine, you will be *ministering* to patients." I began to pray for patients, seeking God's pathway to healing in the supernatural realm as well as in the natural realm.

Over the years we have witnessed how God miraculously uses both supernatural and natural pathways to heal patients and to demonstrate His marvelous healing and saving power.

I know what God has done in my life, and I know what God has done in the lives of our patients. He can do the same in yours. He has a unique pathway to healing for you! He is the Lord, who heals you (Exodus 15:26); by His stripes you are healed (Isaiah 53:5).

Linda and I are standing with you as you seek God's pathway to healing for a healthy heart and cardiovascular system.

If you do not know Jesus Christ as your personal Lord and Savior, I invite you to pray this prayer and ask Jesus into your life:

> *Lord Jesus, I invite you into my life as my Lord and Savior. I repent of my past sins. I ask you to forgive me. Thank you for shedding your blood on the cross to*

cleanse me from my sin and to heal me. I receive your gift of everlasting life and surrender all to you. Thank you, Jesus, for saving me. Amen.

ABOUT THE AUTHOR

Reginald B. Cherry, M.D., did his premed at Baylor University, graduated from the University of Texas Medical School, and has practiced diagnostic and preventive medicine for more than twenty-five years. His work in medicine has been recognized and honored by the city of Houston and by President George W. Bush when he was governor of Texas.

Dr. Cherry and his wife, Linda, a clinical nurse who has worked with Dr. Cherry and his patients during the past two and a half decades, now host the popular television program *The Doctor and the Word*, which has a potential viewing audience of 90 million homes weekly. They also publish a monthly medical newsletter and produce topical audiocassette teachings, pocket books, and booklets. Dr. Cherry is author of the bestselling books *The Doctor and the Word*, *The Bible Cure*, and *Healing Prayer*.

RESOURCES AVAILABLE FROM REGINALD B. CHERRY MINISTRIES, INC.

Books

Prayers That Heal: Faith-Building Prayers When You Need a Miracle

Combining the wisdom of more than twenty-five years of medical practice and the revelation of God's Word, Dr. Cherry provides the knowledge you need to pray effectively against diabetes, cancer, heart disease, eye problems, hypoglycemia, and fifteen other common afflictions that rob you of your health.

Healing Prayer

A fascinating in-depth look at the vital link between spiritual and physical healing. Dr. Cherry presents actual case histories of people healed through prayer, plus the latest information on herbs, vitamins, and supplements that promote vibrant health. This is sound information needed to keep you healthy—mind, soul, and body.

God's Pathway to Healing: Bone Health

Bone mass loss and osteoporosis affect more than 34 million Americans today, and statistics indicate that these numbers will continue to grow dramatically in the decades to come. Though bone disease affects four times the number of women as men, the men who suffer from its complications are often twice as likely to die from them as are women. None of us has room to ignore this debilitating ailment; we all need to do what we can now to either prevent or reverse its effects. In this pocket book, Dr. Cherry shares with readers the things they can do, no matter their age, to strengthen bones and immensely reduce the risks of bone mass loss that results in fractures that can rob us of the quality of life God promised us, if not take life from us altogether. This is a book for all ages and both sexes, as building strong bones is an issue all of us need to address.

God's Pathway to Healing: Diabetes

Diabetes is reaching epidemic proportions as 17 million Americans now face the disease—more than one-third of them not even aware that they have it—and another one million a year will develop it. Some statistics suggest that by the year 2025, one in four Americans will have diabetes. The severe complications of diabetes also give us reason for concern, since it more than triples the risk of death for young adults who acquire it. However, God has a pathway both for prevention and healing of this proliferating disease. In this pocket book, Dr. Cherry outlines the lifestyle changes to prevent and control diabetes as well as the best medications and natural alternatives for reducing its threat to our overall health. This is a book no one can afford to miss, as diabetes most likely affects at least one person you know or love.

God's Pathway to Healing: Digestion

Dr. Cherry discusses keys to a naturally healthy digestive system, including better digestion and absorption of food, proper elimination of waste, and the place of "good" bacteria. He points readers toward better eating habits and natural nutritional supplements to improve digestion.

God's Pathway to Healing: Heart

Heart disease kills twice as many people as all the various forms of cancer combined, and more than half of the body of Christ dies of coronary artery or cardiovascular diseases. However, there are things that you can do to remain free of heart disease. An incredible wealth of research in recent years has been done on natural extracts and foods that will feed this life-sustaining muscle and keep it strong and healthy. When these nutrients are combined with faith, prayer, and God's Word, you will find yourself on God's pathway to healing and a healthy heart.

God's Pathway to Healing: Herbs That Heal

Learn the truth about common herbal remedies and discover the possible side effects of each. Discover which herbs can help treat symptoms of insomnia, arthritis, heart problems, asthma, and many other conditions. Read this book and determine if herbs are part of God's pathway to healing for you.

God's Pathway to Healing: The Immune System

We are truly fearfully and wonderfully made, and part of that amazing creation is something God built into us to keep us all healthy for life: our immune system. In this insightful pocket book, Dr. Cherry explains the basic function of this "everyday miracle," which even medical science has yet to fully understand, as well as steps we can take to keep it strong and balanced so that it will do what God designed it to do: "Keep sickness from the midst of us" (Exodus 23:25).

God's Pathway to Healing: Joints and Arthritis

Painful joints and arthritis do not have to be part of aging, Dr. Cherry says. Recent medical breakthroughs show that natural substances can relieve pain and inflammation and slow or prevent cartilage loss.

God's Pathway to Healing: Memory and Mental Acuity

As the baby-boomer generation ages, we are facing more problems with mental function than ever before. Whether because of age-related memory loss, poor nutrition, or air pollutants, many are aware of a lesser capacity to think clearly and/or to concentrate. People of all ages need new information about how to keep their minds healthy and strong. In this pocket book, Dr. Cherry addresses these concerns in a straightforward and easy-to-understand manner that can help those facing such ailments as depression, attention-deficit hyperactivity disorder (ADHD), migraine headaches, Alzheimer's disease, or other concerns associated with brain function. This book may well be God's key for you to a healthy memory and a sharp, focused mind.

God's Pathway to Healing: Menopause

This small book is full of helpful advice for women who are going through what can be a very stressful time of life. Find out what foods, supplements, and steps lead to a pathway of healing for menopause and perimenopause.

God's Pathway to Healing: Prostate

This pocket book is packed with enlightening insights for men who are searching for ways to prevent prostate cancer or who have actually been diagnosed with the disease. Discover how foods, plant-derived natural supplements, and a change in diet can be incorporated into your life to help you find a pathway to healing for prostate disease.

God's Pathway to Healing: Vision

Macular degeneration, cataracts, vision degeneration due to complications of diabetes, and other eye conditions can be slowed or prevented. Dr. Cherry discusses herbs that are helpful and nutritional changes people can make to keep vision strong.

God's Pathway to Healing: Vitamins and Supplements

With the growing number of supplements and multivitamins on the market today, it is difficult to know what to take and when and how to avoid taking more than is needed or in combinations that could be harmful. This easy-to-follow pocket book is a tremendous reference for anyone desiring to stay healthy in this age when new diseases seem to be discovered more often than ever before. This book could be the key to discovering the miraculous power God has unlocked through natural extracts and nutritional supplements to keep us healthy to the end of our days.

Dr. Cherry's Little Instruction Book for Health and Healing

Easy-to-read information about healthy habits, natural remedies, and nutritional guidance. Biblical principles for supernatural healing, prayers, and Scripture remind us that God's desire is that we be healthy. This is a helpful small volume for readers familiar with Dr. Cherry's work and a great introduction for those who are new to his ministry.

The Bible Cure (now in paperback)

Dr. Cherry presents hidden truths from the Bible taken from ancient dietary health laws, how Jesus anointed with natural substances to heal, and how to activate faith through prayer for health and healing. This book validates scientific medical research by using it to prove God's original health plan.

The Doctor and the Word
(now in paperback)

Dr. Cherry shows how God has a pathway to healing for you. Jesus healed instantaneously and supernaturally, while other healings involved a process. Discover how the manifestation of your healing can come about by seeking His ways.

Dr. Cherry's Study Guides, Volume 2
(bound volume)

Receive thirty valuable resource study guides from topics Dr. Cherry has taught on the Trinity Broadcasting Network (TBN) program *The Doctor and the Word*.

Basic Nutrient Support

Dr. Cherry has developed a daily nutrient supplement that is the simplest to take and yet the most complete supplement available today. Protect your body daily with more than sixty natural substances that fight cancer, heart disease, and many other problems. Call Natural Alternatives at (800)339-5952 to place your order. Please mention service code "BN30" when ordering. (Or order through the company's Web site: *www.AbundantNutrition.com*.)

Cardiovascular Support

Because of its prevalence today, we all need to be concerned about heart disease. To help you get the nutrients you need to keep your heart healthy and strong, Dr. Cherry has developed *Cardiovascular Support*, a powerful combination of nutrients and herbs that support all aspects of cardiovascular function. Call Natural Alternatives at (800)339-5952 to place your order. Please mention service code "BN30" when ordering.

> Reginald B. Cherry Ministries, Inc.
> P.O. Box 27711
> Houston, TX 77227-7711
> 1-888-DRCHERRY

BECOME A PATHWAY TO HEALING PARTNER

We invite you to become a pathway partner. We ask you to stand with us in prayer and financial support as we provide new programs, resources, books, pocket books, and a unique, one-of-a-kind monthly newsletter.

Our monthly "Pathway to Healing Partner Newsletter" sorts through the confusion about health and healing. In it, Dr. Cherry shares sensible, biblical, and medical steps you can take to get well. Every issue points you to your pathway to healing. Writing from a Christian physician's Bible-based point of view, Dr. Cherry talks about nutrition and health, how to pray for specific diseases, updates on the latest medical research, Linda's own recipes for healthy eating, and questions and answers about issues you need to know about.

In addition, we'll provide you with Dr. Cherry and Linda's ministry calendar, broadcast schedule, resources for better living, and special monthly offers.

This newsletter is available to you as you partner with the Cherrys through prayer and monthly financial support to help expand this God-given ministry. Pray today about responding with a monthly contribution of $10 or more. Call or write to the address on the following page to find out how you can receive this valuable information.

Become a Pathway partner today by writing:

Reginald B. Cherry Ministries, Inc.
P.O. Box 27711
Houston, TX 77227-7711
Visit our Web site:
www.drcherry.org
1-888-DRCHERRY

This page is a continuation of the copyright page.

Unless otherwise indicated, Scripture quotations are from the *King James Version* of the Bible.

Scripture quotations marked NKJV are taken from the *New King James Version of the Bible*. Copyright ©1979, 1980, 1982 by Thomas Nelson, Inc. Used by permission. All rights reserved.

Scripture quotations marked NLT are from *The Holy Bible, New Living Translation*, copyright ©1996. Used by permission of Tyndale House Publishers, Inc., Wheaton, Illinois, 60189. All rights reserved.